YO-DKE-374

List Your Self for Pregnancy

Other Books by Ilene Segalove

List Your Self
(with Paul Bob Velick)
Unwritten Letters

Other Books by Gareth Esersky
Please Read This for Me

List Your Self for Pregnancy

Listmaking as the Way to Self-Discovery for the Mother-to-Be

Ilene Segalove and Gareth Esersky

**Andrews McMeel
Publishing**
Kansas City

> The LIST YOUR SELF book series and calendars are the creation of Ilene Segalove and Paul Bob Velick. These listmaking tools invite the reader to become the writer, offering an interactive approach to self-discovery.

List Your Self for Pregnancy copyright © 1999 by Ilene Segalove and Gareth Esersky. All rights reserved. Printed in the United States of America. No part of this book may be used or reproduced in any manner whatsoever without written permission except in the case of reprints in the context of reviews. For information, write Andrews McMeel Publishing, an Andrews McMeel Universal company, 4520 Main Street, Kansas City, Missouri 64111.

www.andrewsmcmeel.com

99 00 01 02 03 RDC 10 9 8 7 6 5 4 3 2 1

ISBN 0-8362-8181-0

Design by Holly Camerlinck

ATTENTION: SCHOOLS AND BUSINESSES

Andrews McMeel books are available at quantity discounts with bulk purchase for educational, business, or sales promotional use. For information, please write to: Special Sales Department, Andrews McMeel Publishing, 4520 Main Street, Kansas City, Missouri 64111.

To Charlotte, Zeke, and Amelia

Contents

Acknowledgments ix
Introduction 1

• one •
Yourself 7

• two •
Your Partner 27

• three •
Your Baby 43

• four •
Daily Life 57

• five •
The Birth 77

• six •
After the Delivery 99

Notes 116

Acknowledgments

The authors would like to express a heartfelt thanks to our terrific editor Chris Schillig and the Andrews McMeel sales force who made *List Your Self* such a success; the readers of *List Your Self*; Jean Zevnik and our design team; Carol Mann, whose agency represents and encourages us; and, of course, the remarkable parents and children—including our own—whose lives, experiences, and expertise inform these lists and enlighten the soul of this book.

Introduction

Self-knowledge is always worth pursuing—getting to know what makes us tick, how we think, who we really are. But there are certain turning points in our lives that ask us to pay closer attention. Your pregnancy is definitely one of those unique and remarkable experiences. *List Your Self for Pregnancy* gives you the opportunity to dive in and discover more about yourself on your journey from early pregnancy through the delivery of your baby. So many changes are going on right now; so many questions and revelations emerge. Since pregnancy has a real beginning, middle, and end, it's the perfect time to chronicle your thoughts. *List Your Self for Pregnancy* provides you with one hundred inspirational list suggestions and plenty of room to jot down and keep track of what's going on during this extraordinary time of your life.

Pregnancy begs to be listed. There are so many things to do, so many things to consider. As you prepare to greet your new baby, you need to handle all kinds of issues you may never have had to grapple with before. Your body is changing. Your emotions are changing. Your relationship to your mate, your family, and your home are being redefined. Important medical choices for your delivery need to be made. Boys' and girls' names float around your mind. You may feel it more difficult to concentrate at work. Daily life isn't quite as simple as it used to be. A torrent of possibilities, both delightful and sometimes terrifying, spin inside you every moment. Nothing is the same. Often you may feel overwhelmed.

List Your Self for Pregnancy is a safe haven from the whirlwind of your busy life. It's a place to take time out, if only for a few minutes, to rejuvenate and renew yourself. Listing is a simple form of journaling and *List Your Self for Pregnancy* is a guided journal that helps you get a handle on some of the physical, psychological, and pragmatic challenges you may be experiencing right now. It gives you the chance to capture important insights that might slip away simply by asking you to fill in the blanks. In so doing, it encourages you to cultivate a deeper relationship with your pregnant self. And it's an easy way to nurture yourself and regain your focus for the days ahead.

List Your Self for Pregnancy soothes your mind and soul. It is also a great way to organize your thoughts into neat categories during a time that you may feel more distracted than usual. Since this is a period in your life that you will want to remember in some detail, *List Your Self for Pregnancy* covers an array of topics that speak to the aspects of your pregnancy you'll want to chronicle: yourself, your partner, your baby, daily life, the birth, and after the delivery. The lists you make will document your pregnancy, from the practical to the profound. Consider the following list suggestion, from Chapter Two: Your Partner: "List all the rational reasons you've both come up with for having a baby." Now that's a list you have probably made a hundred times in your mind. Writing it down clarifies your commitment and actually may make you feel rather proud of yourself.

- It's the next step in our growth as a couple
- Joy
- To grow as an individual with this universal experience
- To give and give
- To stop being so selfish and focus on something outside of myself
- To continue the family lines on both sides
- To give our first child a sibling

Putting pen to paper and expressing yourself will give you a sense of connection to your deepest inner voice. Rereading your list can remind you of what's really important, especially if you sometimes find yourself a little lost or out of sorts. If you forget what it's all about in the midst of daily confusion or chaos, sit down and list your self. You'll find you'll be back on track in no time.

Introduction

Here is a seemingly lighthearted list idea: List all the great moms in your life.

- My own mom, until I turned fourteen, that is
- The YMCA camp director's wife who had three kids and then at forty-three had another one and did the best Christmases ever
- The schoolteacher who lived next door and raised two very handsome, polite, and intelligent sons
- My Russian grandmother who could knit, read the newspaper, cook, give advice, listen to the radio, and teach piano all at once and made the best doughnuts in New Hampshire
- Harriet Nelson, *Leave it to Beaver*'s mom, Jane Wyatt on *Father Knows Best* (it goes on and on)
- Anastasia Gianakopoulos, mother of three girls, and a widow, who taught me all about babies and how to cook a perfect chicken

This list may seem insignificant, at first glance. But once you really examine the names and faces from your past that show up in your mind, you might think twice. There's a lot of information in here. These women may have been part of the reason you chose to be a mom in the first place!

Some of the lists in *List Your Self for Pregnancy* will inspire you to dip into your memory bank, to revisit the pieces of your life that really made a difference. Some of the lists will encourage you to cultivate a deeper connection with your own truth, a truth that hasn't had the chance to be spoken or articulated . . . yet.

List how you think your partner will be a good parent.

- He is fiercely loyal.
- He can be so funny and will laugh with the child.
- He will teach the child so much, from how to make jokes to how to fish.

- He is very protective of me.
- He has a great capacity to love and teach and play.
- He shares the same ideals I do.
- He wants to be a good parent and is committed to raising him or her well.

Pregnancy is such a unique slice of your life. The woman you are now lives inside this special time frame. After you deliver your baby you may forget some of the wonderful and even amusing revelations you had. How about this one: List how you look in a bathing suit or leotard . . . for posterity's sake . . . .

- Like a giant egg with appendages
- Like a bobbing pool toy
- Like from the rear I should wear a WIDE LOAD sign
- Like Mrs. Tweedledum or Tweedledee
- Hard, strong, and immovable
- Like a boulder with tiny feet
- *Very* pregnant

List Your Self for Pregnancy is easy and fun to use. You may wish to open the book up randomly to whatever list shows up and fill in the blanks. So you simply flip open the book and there is "List all the unique, intriguing baby names you love that you know you can't use." Suddenly Ignatious and Sunshine come to mind. Or on a more serious note, say today you are thinking a lot about your delivery. Find the appropriate chapter, read through the list suggestions, and take some time to consider how you feel. There are plenty of provocative list suggestions that will help you evaluate and chronicle your concerns. Or you may flip through the book and scan the lists on the top of each page until one jumps out at you and begs to be listed: "List the stuff you need to put in 'the Bag' to take to the hospital for the new baby . . . for yourself and your birth partner." You've been thinking about this for months now, but just haven't been able to jot it down. As you look at the list suggestion

Introduction

you find yourself, well, listing. It comes naturally. And your answers pour out easily.

- a telephone credit card or number so I can call everyone
- camera and film
- my own pillows and pillowcases
- a bottle of champagne?

Write your answers quickly or slowly. It doesn't matter how, just make sure you are as honest as you can be. Keep your answers personal. And writing whatever comes to mind first is always a good idea. Usually it is the truest expression of the real you. Try not to get stuck in your head, thinking what the "right" answer is. There are no "right" answers. This is your book, a portrait of who you are right now. That's the beauty and power of *List Your Self for Pregnancy*. It is like a snapshot of the unique woman you are at this wondrous juncture in time. Years from now this book will be a meaningful and informative nine-month time capsule and a legacy of the here and the now. And when you share it with your child one day, it will reflect the vibrant passion and truth that is you . . . today.

You can *List Your Self for Pregnancy* wherever you are. It's the perfect thing to do when you are waiting at the doctor's office, when you wake up, or before you go to sleep. It's also great to dip into when you are tired or upset. It will give you a focus, clear your head, and may even make you smile.

Your pregnancy is a great time to pay extra attention. The archaic root of "list" means to listen to. Listen to yourself and explore your depths. Jump in and document this memorable and momentous piece of your life. Take out a pen, settle into *List Your Self for Pregnancy*, and come home to yourself.

• one •

Yourself

*L*ist the way you felt when you first saw the image of your baby on the ultrasound monitor.

Yourself

*L*ist what makes you cry, or other examples of "hormone madness."

List Your Self for Pregnancy

*L*ist *how being pregnant is different than you ever thought it would be.*

List all the things that show up in your dreams that amaze you.

List Your Self for Pregnancy

List what you look like in a bathing suit.

Yourself

List the ways you feel about your age and being pregnant.

*L*ist some of the first thoughts you had when you found out you were pregnant. (*N*ow, don't censor.)

Yourself

List who you told you were pregnant and when (what month).

List Your Self for Pregnancy

List all your favorite clothes you've put out to pasture for a while.

Yourself

List the things you do to make yourself look pretty now that you're pregnant.

List Your Self for Pregnancy

List the physical changes in your body that you find fascinating, although not necessarily attractive.

Yourself

List your best qualities you hope you'll pass on to your child.

List the odd habits you've developed since you've been pregnant.

$\mathcal{L}$ist *what you feel you have free license to do now that you're pregnant.*

List what you like best about how pregnancy affects the way you view the world, yourself, and others.

*L*ist all the weird cravings you have noticed lately.

List Your Self for Pregnancy

*L*ist all the things you're doing (the foods you're eating, the vitamins you're taking) to help you have a healthier pregnancy.

Yourself

List your most profound and private revelations about the joy and miracle of being pregnant.

• two •

Your Partner

List Your Self for Pregnancy

*L*ist how your sex life has changed since you've been pregnant.

Your Partner

*L*ist all the rational reasons you've both come up with for having a baby.

List Your Self for Pregnancy

*L*ist all the irrational reasons you've both given for wanting a child.

Your Partner

List the names your significant other calls you now that you are pregnant.

*L*ist how your mate has really "shown up" for you with gifts, kind words, or other encouragement and understanding.

List the joyous moments you've spent celebrating your pregnancy with your mate.

*L*ist all the ways your sleeping patterns and habits have changed to accommodate your pregnancy and your mate.

Your Partner

List all the ways being pregnant has deepened the connection you have with your mate.

List Your Self for Pregnancy

List the crazy ideas your mate has suggested for documenting your childbirth.

Your Partner

List some of the meals your mate has cooked for you day or night.

List some of the recurring fears your mate has expressed.

Your Partner

List the ways you know your partner will be a good parent.

List Your Self for Pregnancy

*L*ist the feelings you've been holding back that you want to tell your partner.

Your Partner

List the things your partner did or said when you announced you were pregnant.

List Your Self for Pregnancy

ℒist your partner's unusual behavior since you have been pregnant (like maybe gaining weight, too).

• three •

Your Baby

*L*ist the responsibilities you feel about bringing a new life into the world.

Your Baby

ℒist all the stuff you've collected for your new baby.

*L*ist *all the new things you need to buy for your baby.*

Your Baby

List all the unique baby names you love that you know you can't use.

List Your Self for Pregnancy

*L*ist your deepest daily fears about your baby's health.

Your Baby

$\mathcal{L}$ist all the things you love about babies.

List Your Self for Pregnancy

ℒist how you describe the miracle of actually carrying a life around inside of you.

Your Baby

List the superstitions you've heard and maybe even believe about pregnancy.

*L*ist the reasons to know the sex of the baby.

List the reasons not to learn the sex of the baby.

List Your Self for Pregnancy

List the boys' and girls' names that you love.

*L*ist all the odd, spiritual, or maybe ESP-like feelings you've had during pregnancy.

List Your Self for Pregnancy

*L*ist how you feel when you see someone else's baby.

• four •

Daily Life

List Your Self for Pregnancy

List how your parents treat you differently now that you're pregnant.

List all the ways the world has responded to your pregnancy.

List the daily acts that you used to take for granted that are now a little tougher to do.

Daily Life

*L*ist the books you want to read or buy (including another copy of this book for a friend).

List Your Self for Pregnancy

ℒist all the ways your mom is involved in your pregnancy, good and bad.

Daily Life

List your fears about how your coworkers and clients may react to your pregnancy.

List Your Self for Pregnancy

List all the good advice you've received from other mothers.

List the maternal leave benefits you wish your insurance included or your employer offered.

List Your Self for Pregnancy

*L*ist the good stuff about looking pregnant.

*L*ist *the typical responses people have when you tell them you are pregnant.*

List Your Self for Pregnancy

List what you pretended life would be like when you were pregnant compared to what it is really like.

Daily Life

*L*ist how you feel when people want to touch your pregnant belly.

List Your Self for Pregnancy

List all the special—and sometimes embarrassing—ways people treat you now that they know you are pregnant.

*L*ist the magazines and books you read and the shows you watch because you are pregnant.

List Your Self for Pregnancy

List all the junk, furniture, and stuff you have to get rid of to make room for the baby.

Daily Life

*L*ist how you'll have to babyproof the house.

List Your Self for Pregnancy

*L*ist the ways you have to schedule doctor's appointments and other baby-related responsibilities around work.

*L*ist what you've given up now that you're pregnant.

• five •

The Birth

List Your Self for Pregnancy

*L*ist the reasons to have drugs during labor and delivery.

The Birth

List the reasons for a natural, drug-free childbirth.

List Your Self for Pregnancy

*L*ist what you fear you will never get to do again after the baby comes.

The Birth

List the people in your Lamaze or birth preparation class, their addresses, phone numbers, and due dates.

_____

_____

_____

_____

_____

_____

_____

_____

_____

_____

_____

_____

_____

_____

_____

_____

_____

_____

_____

_____

_____

_____

List the questions you need to ask potential pediatricians.

The Birth

List how you visualize the ideal birth, including how you go into labor, what you feel, and how the doctor/midwife and your partner respond to you.

*L*ist the questions you think may be "stupid" but you must know the answers to anyway.

List the questions to ask when you take the tour of the maternity wing or birthing center.

*L*ist the questions you want to ask your mother about being pregnant.

The Birth

List the questions you will never ask your mother about being pregnant.

List what you want to know about your own birth.

The Birth

*L*ist the good things about a birthing center.

List the benefits of giving birth in a hospital.

The Birth

*L*ist *your feelings about having a C-section.*

List Your Self for Pregnancy

List what your obstetrician or midwife has told you that you just cannot believe.

The Birth

List your greatest fears about your delivery.

List all the worries you have about what might be wrong with your baby.

The Birth

*L*ist all the scary things people tell you that might go wrong during the birth.

List Your Self for Pregnancy

*L*ist the stuff you need to put in "the Bag" to take to the hospital for the new baby.

The Birth

*L*ist the stuff you need to put in "the Bag" to take to the hospital for yourself and your birth partner.

six

After the Delivery

List Your Self for Pregnancy

*L*ist all the great mothers from your life whose behavior will be an inspiration for you.

List the way you feel when putting your baby in the crib for the very first time.

List Your Self for Pregnancy

*L*ist all the fears you have about how your life will never be the same.

List all the things you can't wait to do again after you deliver your baby.

List how this pregnancy is different from your earlier one(s).

After the Delivery

*L*ist the people to whom you will send birth announcements.

List Your Self for Pregnancy

List all the baby stuff you think is ridiculous or a waste of money.

List the child-care agencies or friendly contacts you have for finding a permanent child-care giver.

*L*ist *the questions to ask when interviewing a potential child-care person.*

List the people—friends, family, coworkers—whom you can count on to help you after the baby arrives.

List Your Self for Pregnancy

List the terms of endearment you'll want to call your new infant.

After the Delivery

List the baby clothes and basic infant equipment you will definitely need as soon as you come home.

List the baby clothes or equipment you can borrow and from whom.

List the pros and cons of breast-feeding and your concerns.

List Your Self for Pregnancy

*L*ist the phone numbers of the LaLeche League, their support people, and the "new mothers' hotline."

After the Delivery

List the ways you and your mate will celebrate the birth of your new baby.

Notes

Notes

Notes